Going Straight

Going Straight

Living with Ankylosing Spondylitis-
A Laugh a minute!

Alan Greaves

authorHOUSE®

AuthorHouse™
1663 Liberty Drive
Bloomington, IN 47403
www.authorhouse.com
Phone: 1-800-839-8640

First published by AuthorHouse   11/04/2011

ISBN: 978-1-4567-8305-1 (sc)

Printed in the United States of America

Preface

My wonderful friends, Colin and Mig, suggested that I should write my story of a life spent in company with Ankylosing Spondylitis, (AS). Colin, believing that I should leave it for my family as a memoir, Mig seeing it more as a source of information for the Spondylitic community.

Of course, I am delighted to recount the tale. I do love talking about it all because I think, that in the battle against it I was one of life's lucky ones, but a story about AS? Where does one begin?

I think then that it is important not to bore ever onward about the dry topic of an unpleasant illness but rather to talk about my life and only include AS when it included itself in my everyday affairs, unfortunately its interference was/is almost perpetual.

What is Ankylosing Spondylitis?

Ankylosing Spondylitis is a form of chronic inflammation of the spine and the underline:[sacroiliac joints]. The sacroiliac joints are located in the low back where the sacrum (the bone directly above the tailbone) meets the iliac bones (bones on either side of the upper buttocks). Chronic inflammation in these areas causes pain and stiffness in and around the spine. Over time, chronic spinal inflammation (**S**pondylitis) can lead to a complete cementing together (fusion) of the vertebrae, a process referred to as **a**nkylosis. Ankylosis leads to loss of mobility of the spine. Ankylosing Spondylitis is also a systemic disease, meaning it can affect other tissues throughout the body. Accordingly, it can cause inflammation in or injury to other joints away from the spine, as well as to other organs, such as the eyes, heart, lungs and kidneys.

Another definition is rather more straightforward than the foregoing. It is about what AS means daily to the sufferer. These few words say it all:

Spinal Disease
Chronic
Progressive
Pain
Lassitude
Fusion
Deformity
Loss of function
Threats to well being of eyes and heart
Utter misery

Lots more pain
Perpetuity

My grateful thanks to my friends: Colin Tuck for the trolley sketch and my fellow spondylitic, Melinda Page for the spinal drawing and her assistance in compiling this book.

Ankylosing Spondylitis–AS

A twist in the tail-Bone!

I always look at it in terms of my height:

A strapping 6 feet 5 inches

Years of AS reduced me to 5 feet 9 inches

Surgeons took me back to 6 feet 2 inches

Sadly, I am 'on the bend' again but still manage just over 6 feet.

Part 1

*I had a job in a circus as a lion tamer. Well, to be truthful, I was selling orange juice
and popcorn but they did have a lion! That was when I was still at school and when
I met Mary Bacynski, my first love, my first kiss, then her Dad came home but that is
another story . . .*

—One—

THE BARE BONES

I enlisted in the Nottingham City Police Force.

I had had some twinges in my body for a while but worried little about
them and thought they would go away.

Because I was new, novice like, I was first put on night duty. As with all
young policemen it was thought that I could not do a lot of harm in an
empty city centre while at the same time easing me into the job. This was
a fairly standard practice at the time. The shift began at 10:00 pm and was
to end at 6:00 am.

At 4:00 am I could barely walk. I was riddled with pain, most severe in
hips and thighs. I mean really severe! My right leg felt as if a thick wire was
wrapped around it with someone pulling either end, applying all possible
force to the stranglehold the wire had upon me.

I presumed that it was because I had been walking all night, I was new to the job and the physical demands were not what I was yet used to. In a short time I was sure that I would be hardened up and fit for purpose. I daren't complain about it; being a policeman was a dream I had long cherished, so I kept quiet, not wanting anything to 'queer my employment pitch'. In fact I didn't get used to the pain, I didn't harden up. Over one year later the pains were worse, spreading. Around eighteen months into my service I was forced to take time off.

"Hold up, hold up young Greaves, we don't take time off sick."

The nine feet tall sergeant, who arrived at my home ten minutes after I had reported my regretful, yet unavoidable absence, was unimpressed.

"Out of bed let me see you walking around."

In that moment I came fully to understand what was meant by 'Spondylitic' morning stiffness. I could not get out of bed. Pain was remorseless, extreme. I had never known it as strong as this.

The Sergeant, well, he inevitably considered me a faker. He insisted that the doctor be called. His concern was to show that there was evidence of his effort to get me back to work but also to exonerate him from that failed attempt; to have an official note proving that I actually, really was poorly. My persisting agony was to him, of little consequence.

Dr White arrived. He straight away knelt on my bed and bounced around a bit. His 'trampolining' prowess did nothing for my state of mind or my spine and scored a resounding minus in regard to the hoped for reduction in my pain quotient. These antics did however, lay bare the bedsteads failings; it was quickly found guilty as charged of being soft and no good for the improvement of a little backache. I must say that I thought the 'Little Backache' diagnosis slightly wide of the mark! I was prescribed co-codamol, three to be taken with food each day. The bed, sadly, had no such luck and was to be sent for surgery, a mattressectomy imminent.

—Two—

CASING THE JOINT

Life in the police, my dream job, became more and more difficult. I began to believe that the pain would never end, that it would always be there and yet, in my heart I knew that one day it would be ok.

How wrong can one be?

One night, I was severely beaten by 4 men in a cinema; knocked backwards through a row of cinema seating (the old fashioned kind). I took the back of one seat off with my spine, propelled thus by a thrilling right hook that, had it been aimed at anyone else, would have been worthy of high praise! At the time, mind you, my face hurt so much that I didn't notice my spine pain. I have often wondered if this event might have been the trigger to my aggressive AS but know really that I had endured spondylitic pain before this incident, thus rather squashing the 'triggered by trauma' theory.

I worked in a boisterous city centre and was involved in a few fracas, with me usually coming off worse. Aggression seems to abound in city centres. Even in the 1960's when times were thought less violent than now, it was ever present; booze fuelled usually, sometimes very ugly and unpleasant, occasionally fatal.

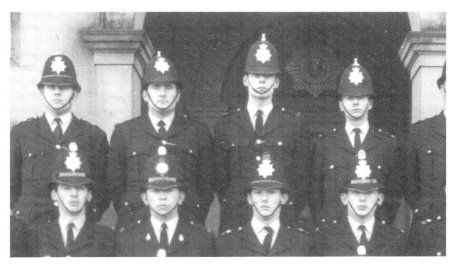

Alan Greaves—Top row—3rd from left. The only one, I am pleased to say, that wore his chin strap in the correct manner.

I had to leave the Police Force. The job that I had cosseted since early school days slipped away from me.

I was in unexplained pain all of the time. It was unbearable. I was a liability in my job, which by nature could, and often did, become very physical.

By now I suffered knife-like pains in the back of my hips. The spinal/hips intersection was a continual, agonising ache. My thighs were weak and it was always painful to walk for longish periods. Medications seemed to make no discernible impression upon the symptoms of whatever this mystery illness was. I became depressed because I was never pain free and I didn't know why. I had noticed, more worryingly, that the pain was now beginning to occur slightly higher up in the spine. It was an effort to bend and I was desperately tired most of the time. Work was a real effort.

Time went by. I took a succession of jobs, all unsatisfactory, all disappointing. Visits to hospitals became more frequent; more necessary. Eventually, I spent time undergoing tests at the City Hospital in Nottingham. I was in real trouble, by now incapable of doing much that was of use!

At home, in an endeavour to gain some level of relief, I was getting up at night turning on the gas fire, lying on my side with my back as close to the fire as it was possible to do without searing the skin. Heat helped a little in those days or at least it replaced one unpleasant sensation with another slightly less unpleasant one. Very hot baths would be rather like lying before the fire and provide a modicum of temporary relief.

Following the hospital tests, I was prescribed Phenylbutazone, an anti-inflammatory drug. I took this for many years. It did no good, only causing other problems which, like Mary Bacynski, do not belong in this particular tale.

I was under the care of Consultant Rheumatologist, Dr. Sam James. There is now a ward at the City Hospital which is named after him. By now I had endured four years of agony on a moment by moment basis. Dr. James eventually told me, following the fearsome, pressing demand for answers he received from one of my wives, that I had a rare disease called Ankylosing Spondylitis. He simplified the description in two ways:

1. Arthritis of the spine
2. Young man's Arthritis

He told me that it could be unpleasant but that it would burn itself out after twenty years and all would be well. The answer was still Phenylbutazone, this despite the fact that after taking hundreds of the things, there had been no change.

"Keep Mobile." He said.

Yes, that was right. It was then and still is, in my view, the best advice for spondylitics.

I struggled on in hopeful anticipation of an early burn out, a reprieve perhaps, for some years but it didn't burn out, it didn't get better, only worse and worse and worse . . .

Eventually, resignedly, I arrived at the moment, the seminal one, the one to which I had resisting yet inexorably been dragged, there at last to accept AS, as my given lot and in so doing, being shown not one whit of compassion by the victor.

I knew now that this wasn't going away. AS would always be a part of me and all the days of my life to come would be horribly despoiled by this thing.

Because knowledge can be strength! I knew then that it was time for me, despite AS, to try to regain control of my life and live it as best I could, despite this debilitating condition. How best to do this? Well, why not try to do all of the things that AS wouldn't let me do! So I went to work on construction sites, a mistake no doubt, for here the damage to my spine was exacerbated, but I had to live, I had to work, I had somehow to keep going.

My reward for these efforts, as if Ankylosing Spondylitis had not already damaged me enough, was that it now began in earnest. It struck me, that the disease had decided to stop 'pussyfooting' around with me and to do the job properly! It was now that I realised that my movement was becoming restricted. I continued to endure the remorselessness of awful pain, gagging, lung restricting, felling.

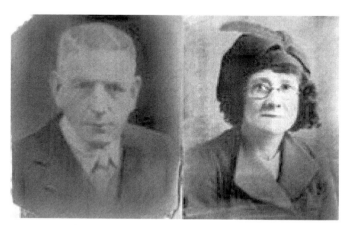

My grandparents: John Byron Greaves and Florence Greaves.

John Byron, it seems, was a spondylitic too. My mother describes him as severely stooped, evidence for the hereditary nature of this awful disease. Unfortunately I never met them.

I once rescued Norman Wisdom, who had locked himself out of his car (a white Rover) when he did a show at the Theatre Royal, Nottingham. I remember thinking to impress him with a well delivered joke:

"Norman, isn't it a lovely day for pouring custard down your mother-in-law's knickers?"

"You'll go far" he said.

—Three—

BACK ON FORM?

By now the disease had spread to ribs and upper spine. In addition, I now had the pleasure of terrible spinal stiffness in the morning, so extreme that it usually took two hours after rising from a nights sleep (if such were ever the case) before movement was possible and sufficient to enable the mobility required for walking, driving and so on.

The pains were progressing along the spine, ever upwards. It felt as if baby elephants in stiletto heels were dancing on my rear ribcage; finding without fail, each and every delicate area and bearing heavily down upon them. I had nerve jangling pains in the ribs, where they attach to the spine. An almost permanent sensation, like that of a metal strap clamped cruelly around the chest, front and back, reminiscent of some medieval torture, ever tightening leaving ribs begging for relief.

In short, I was now affected entirely from just above the knees, almost to shoulder level. I prayed daily for the promised yet elusive 'burn out'.

Four

Put Your Back Into It

Life for me, certainly between the ages of 21 to 35, was a living hell. These were the years of my youth, a youth which was utterly besmirched by this grim interloper. I did not, could not do the things that Mr and Mrs Average could do. AS robbed me of those years. Pain was ever present, fusion well under way, following the classic course, starting at the coccyx and steadily creeping up the spine. I rarely went to the doctor or the hospital now because medications were unhelpful. I was over the years, prescribed variously:

> Phenylbutazone
> Co-codamol
> Co-Proxamol
> Indomethacin
> Naprosyn
> Arthrotec
> Diclofenac
> Voltarol
> Brufen
> Ibruprofen

There were many others, the names of which have long since left me.

None worked but then how would I know if they did? Perhaps they did, perhaps the pain would have been even worse without them? It seemed unlikely because to me, it felt as awful as it could possibly be. One of my wives had to fetch me from work one day, the boss had summoned her to appear to collect the staff member whose grunts and sharp intakes of breath were driving away his clientele. I simpered all the way home, all afternoon, all night, not because I am weak but because I had hurt so much for so long and could not envisage an end to it, ever. And yes I did, I thought about it, I thought about the only alternative that I could see to this permanent hellish nightmare of pain.

How, when, would I be able to do it? Who would find me? Would they say I was a weak coward, a waster and deserved nothing more than I got? Anything though, anything was worth considering to escape this bastard of an illness. I didn't, though. Like all AS-ers, somehow and from somewhere, you find the will to go for another day.

That night I walked the estate for hours, anything to try to walk it off or try to forget about it and actually, around about four in the morning, it began to ease.

My son was born soon after this; my wife left me shortly after that!

I next saw Chris (my son) twenty years later. He has some slight indications of AS. We pray that he will escape it.

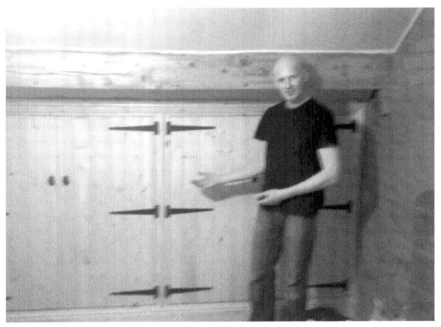

Christopher, my son, showing off my handiwork!

Depressed about losing the police job, no other work seemed appealing. In my life I wanted two things:

1. To be a policeman, and I wasn't.
2. Not to have AS, and I had.

What to do, how to make purposefulness from this mess. I had only one other minor skill, music. Could music save me?

I have never written anything longer than four words before. I find myself in uncharted literary seas, adrift without a paddle, sailing alone and lonely, to whom knows where? Music was the thing.

—Five—

Backing Down

I am a man of passion though not driven by passions, a man with copious draughts of moral outrage and yet not outrageous, some would say not very moral either. My great hero, Beethoven, was a man of passion and enormously gifted. He was a loner, like me.

However (I once was yelled at by a teacher for starting a sentence with the difficult and troubling word 'however'.

"Never start a sentence with a preposition." He cawed, sneering down at me, pompous and smug. I walked off and left him there. I was forty-seven at the time but felt as foolish then as I always had when I was at school.)

He (the teacher) didn't have AS, neither did Beethoven, but both had unseemly long hair! Why they have appeared in this story I don't know, perhaps a subconscious way of chasing away the writers block . . . .

I joined a band in 1974, November. In the end, I played with that band for over ten years; until they got rid of me, mainly because I couldn't play very well! It was more likely because I looked not so good on stage. The deformity was pronounced by now and became exponentially more so throughout those ten years. The sad truth was that I was a poor advertisement for a band that wanted to go out gigging and chasing women. The latter of course appealed not at all to me but I liked playing and the money was handy too. I became all but alcoholic; lost yet another wife; was riddled with AS. Whisky is a good cure, well, a temporary cure perhaps.

My life was falling apart by now. I was laughed at because of the way I looked; mocked because I was always drunk; the one everyone else wanted to take out because all knew there would be a chance of a good laugh at my expense, sometime during the evening.

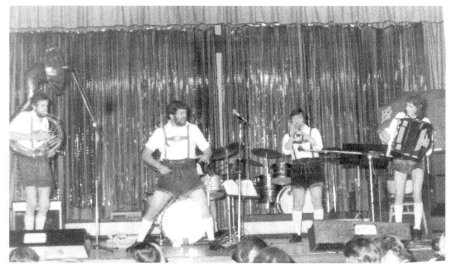

Spot the burgeoning Spondylitic!

I didn't make maintenance payments (alimony) to one of my former beloveds and was twice, whilst on stage, arrested for this. I came to know the particular officer (for it was always the same one) quite well. For his part, he was always as discreet and as pleasant as possible whilst pursuing his duties and he always had a pint that was charged to my account!

Ever my biggest sadness, was not AS, not the booze, not the loss of wives, nor my self respect, but that I was no longer a policeman. Whenever I was marched off to be bailed, I would chat with Bill (that will do for his name) about the police and the job and I would always slip into the conversation,

"I used to be a policeman, you know."

Then the moments of sober propriety, when I would remember what I had been and realise what I now was.

AS was unmoved by my moral decline, my slide into 'failureship'. AS felt, like Bill, that it really ought to do its duty and grind me down that last inch or two, just to make sure that my nose was really jammed hard into the mud. I hurt every moment of every day. When I look back, remarkably, I worked on construction sites by day, played in a band 7 nights a week and then over to the nightclub (The Parkside) where the whisky, for a while at least, made me think I was ok again.

The band residency ended and we finished up 'on the road', 'gigging' at far away places. It is called 'On the road' because that is where you spend almost all of your time; plying the roads and motorways, night and day from one gig to another, trapped in a shoddy van where the band equipment takes pride of place, the players having to squeeze in where they can. Not good for a progressing Spondylitic. Sleep was a rare commodity, so one would squeeze into the van, curl up around a speaker or a guitar case and try to doze. I could never find a comfortable position, so spent my time cramped into a facsimile of a seat and smoked endlessly. I hated being 'on the road'.

I met a girl who was prepared to accept what I had become; she stole my wallet and was never seen again. Another and another and another, always in drink and always in grim realisation of the awakening morning to come; the alcoholic euphoria fading, to be replaced by a depressing, sobering, reality check of my life.

And throughout, AS, good old AS, never let me down; always there to add to the turmoil, to turn the screw, to ratchet up one more notch on the misery-ometer. Then one night, I collapsed.

I was in the band changing room; suddenly I was asleep, there was a brief awakening when a man raked his knuckles along my sternum, it hurt intensely, someone had flatulated; then it was blackness again.

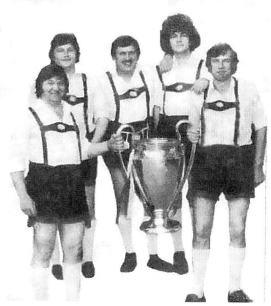

Forest lifted the European Cup. and, back in Nottingham, Karl and the Heidelbergers were ready to hold it high. **JOHN BRUNTON** looks back to 1979, which was also the height of the bierkeller boom

Health to the glory days for Forest — and 'Karl'

The Band

Karl And The Heidelberger's

We were quite famous in the area and quite well known further afield.

Terry—Trumpet, Clive—Drums, Carl—the terrifically good front man, Neil—Keyboards (my brother), and a slightly pre-collapse, bending, drunken bass player—me! 30 years old looking 50!

—Six—

BACK AGAIN

I AWOKE IN HOSPITAL, BROUGHT BACK TO LIFE BY A PRETTY NURSING SISTER PRODDING MY RIBS.

"What is the last thing you remember?"

She repeated it until I could summon a response.

"Happiness." I heard myself saying.

"Oh Great," she said, "He's one of them."

I wasn't sure what one of them was but felt certain that I wasn't one and even if I was one then she had no right to accuse me of being one, which I wasn't and would have refused to be, if I knew what one was or what they did, well I felt a right one! She had turned from a happy bunny into an irritated efficient . . .

"We don't want your sort in here."

I felt like a criminal. I do remember though that her legs were long and sinuous. I was embarrassed too, at being in Accident and Emergency (for I presumed that was where I was), dressed in lederhosen! Yes that's right, Lederhosen. It may seem funny but it wasn't. Well, at least not for the wearer. I have to admit that there seemed to be much mirth in the general area of the trolley upon which I was recumbent.

They tested me for hours and found nothing, not even the AS. Declared me fit and well and said I could go home. So, picture the scene; there I am, in the middle of a huge hospital campus, spondylitically stooped, wearing lederhosen and a white shirt with embroidered front, long socks and red baseball boots. No money, no idea what time it was but knew that I lived miles from where I was. There were many folks milling about and all, it seemed, found me to be an object of interest and amusement . . . . there were no mobile phones then so I asked a nurse if I could use the hospital phone, explaining that I had no money. Yes she said I could.

"You aren't ringing Germany are you?" She chuckled and skipped away.

I managed to raise my brother, another musician, who came and collected me.

This was the first really serious indication perhaps that my time was here, that things had to change, that drinking, working all day and night, sleeping on friend's floors, feeling sorry for myself because my wife had left me and so on was not doing me any good. The brain started to work and to challenge the body, to say, lets try to live a better life than this.

The next day my right knee grew to the size of the Queen Mary. So twenty-four hours later, there I was again, in the hospital having my knee aspirated. Lots of synovial fluid drained off though a needle, barely smaller than Cleopatra's, which was roughly inserted between the kneecap and the bones beneath. Then they admitted me to the ward.

"Oh, why?" I said, "It's only a swollen knee."

"No Alan, it is rather more than a swollen knee."

So, there I was, hospitalised. Not working, no money, alone now. But, for the first time in some years, sober.

—Seven—

BACKED INTO A CORNER

The knee aspiration, now that was an interesting affair. I was hospitalised for a good time on what was euphemistically known then as 'Bed Rest'.

After two weeks they said, go home Alan. I got out of bed and immediately fell onto the floor. I was stooped, seriously stooped. This was the first time that I was aware that my posture had changed. It was a sobering moment. I had noticed stooping before but felt that I could correct it when the pain eased. Now I knew that I couldn't, that this was a permanent state. The pain was there, ever present, the fusion was doing its work, now I was bending forward.

No job to speak of and a drunkard. Something had to change.

The Foreign Legion seemed a good idea at the time, but, even they don't like stooped drunks in the ranks! Cleaning windows was out because I couldn't reach. I had lost the best job ever and was disillusioned with playing because music helped me become a lush. Well, I helped me become a lush but playing put me in the best environment for it. The disease attacked on all sides. No money. A prospect of carrying on as a musician which held the promise of more booze, or giving up the band which would leave me bereft of income.

I lost my home because I didn't keep up the payments and as such was homeless apart from friend's floors. The back of a van, believe it or not, was my bed for some weeks, parked on motorway service stations. I was usually moved on by the police. I was becoming a vagrant, a hobo.

I gained a nickname in the band 'The Maestro'. I wasn't awarded this name for any musical connotation though. Some thought it an appropriate name because of my trick; the trick of wooing a woman every night in order that I might get a bed. Anyone would do, as long as they had a bed and I could sleep. I managed it now and then and was thankful. The back of a van does AS no good. I left the band.

I was fortunate enough to obtain a job in a music shop. I rented a flat using my girlfriend's name. (Yes, I had found a regular girl, I am married to her now!) Suddenly I was warm again, earning a little and the drinking was slowing down, but of course, it is rare that all news is good news. AS had and was progressing at such a rate that I soon realised that I wasn't stooped anymore, I was a human walking stick. My girlfriend didn't seem to mind, she said she liked me as I was, heaven sent words. I changed jobs, I started to work for a hotel (The Royal Moat House International Hotel in Nottingham).

I earned more money here, I became a low level manager and ran a small estates team comprised of carpenters, painters and the like.

One day we were working at the top of a tower scaffold maybe 30 feet up, because by now I was so stooped, I couldn't reach the work above my head, so had to sit on the railings at the side of the tower which gave me an extra two feet height and got me closer to the work.

Idiot that I was and am, I slipped backwards. In desperation and blinding panic, I shot a hand out hoping to get hold of something, thankfully I got hold of a railing and hung on. You see, there is one huge benefit of having AS and useless back muscles, your arms become much more powerful to compensate, because of this I was able to hang on until my friend Jeff, who was up there with me, managed to drag me back up.

It's All Coming Back To Me Now Nurse!

I recovered from my near fatal fall from the scaffold. The hotel fire alarm rang a day or two later. Fire alarms in hotels are a majorly serious issue.

I was the hotel fire officer. I was in the yard when I heard the bells and so I ran toward the staff entrance in order to read the alarm panel and establish where the blaze was. A metal shutter protected the staff entrance but it was in the raised position. In my haste to save all hotel staff and guests from a life threatening false alarm, (we never did have a real fire—thankfully), I continued my dash to the shutter, saw that now, it was on the way down but barely, so 'ducked' under it as I hurried in . . . . well, nearly hurried in, but was belayed by a newly discovered affect of Ankylosing Spondylitis.

I wondered how it was that my eyes saw the shutter descending; my brain adjusted my posture to take me under it as it descended . . . well, nearly, except AS fooled my brain and I was an inch too high as I went under. The next moment, I was crumpled on the floor, blood everywhere and the shutter above me creeping ever lower, heading towards my prone body. My head hurt terribly.

Thankfully, Johnny Ball, a chef and a 'would be' builder friend, (he spent more time in our workshops than in his kitchen), was just inside the shutter; he gripped my arms and pulled me along the floor as the shutter rang out its closing serenade.

Thanks John.

So, off to the hospital once more.

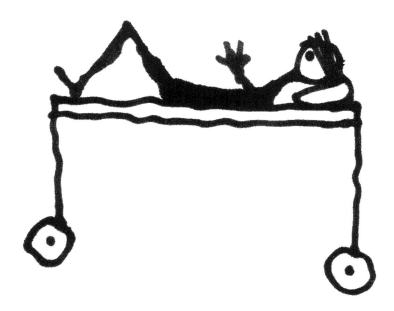

"It's him again."

It was almost a guard of honour as the staff cheered me into A&E, clutching a bath towel sized cotton wool pad to my throbbing head.

Stitched and all ok, I had learned a valuable new lesson. AS interferes with sensory judgements and as such, slow tempo and entering through non-moving shutters might be a better approach to fire fighting. Anyway, I didn't save anyone or anything that day, least of all my now well tarnished tough guy image!

Halfway through the 1980's and I was, by now, really bent forward. A chambermaid who entered a lift that I was in, greeted me beautifully, succinctly,

"Ayup Spastic"

She chortled merrily, clearly pleased with her fine humour.

I was very aware that I looked different, really different and it troubled me. I had always been happy to be tall, despite the discrimination that smaller people seem to have for the tall! Now I was 'quasimodesque', people were laughing and pointing at me. I guessed that they were talking with each other about the crippled maintenance man. I was embarrassed often and usually kept away from the jobs that were adjacent to people.

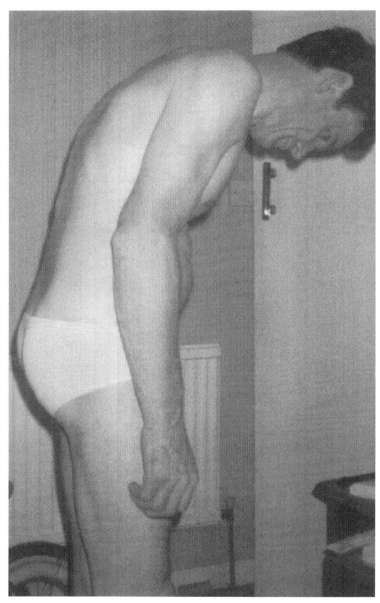

2 years before surgery—no not leaning forward, that was my shape. It was fixed and permanent apart from more forward bending yet to come

Unhappy in some ways with my work, having always aspired to some sort of cerebral role in life I decided to return to college. I was and am a terrible scholar, so this was, for me a brave decision. I was guided really by the knowledge that one day soon AS would make any kind of physical labour difficult, or indeed, impossible and that the bending was increasing at a rate of knots, I decided to try for a qualification in the IPM, yep you got it, an IPM!!!

Oh, you aren't sure??

'Institute of Personnel Management'.

Bernard, my boss,

"No Mr Greaves, don't do that, do teaching."

"What? Mind your own business Bernard."

Yet, as I walked away it struck me. Bernard had sewn a seed, teaching, but teaching ADULTS, I liked the idea.

And so it was that I came to meet DM, a gay midwifery sister, who insisted that she be known as Mel.

Mel gave me the best advice of my life.

Part 2

James Hanratty was the last man to be hanged in England. The execution was as condemned, as was Hanratty. The evidence was flimsy and what there was, seemed to point away from his guilt rather than to it. He was accused of being a car thief but he could not drive. This was the case known as the 'A6 Murder', his family still seek a pardon.

—Nine—

BACK TO THE FUTURE

"We have it to do" said Mel.

She always said it. We had been paired in a mock teaching practice. Well, there were three of us actually, Laura, the other, but she was only on the course because she was having an affair with the lecturer, best not to mention their real names here. In essence the lesson was down to Mel and me. Crime and punishment was the topic, we did a whole thing on James Hanratty, the whys and wherefores. When we had finished, we had persuaded the class that Hanratty should have been acquitted, I still believe it today.

I became firm friends with Mel, a blunt, speak your mind sort of woman.

"Why don't you get your back straightened?" She looked me in the eye.

"Oh they can't do that, there is no procedure."

"Crap." she said, "Go to your doctor, tell him you want surgery, when he says you can't, quote the 'Patient's Charter' at him."

Well, I am not much of a 'quoter' at the best of times, and certainly not to the doctor. I was a child of the age of sitting quietly and speaking only when spoken too, not even then if it were to a Doctor, mother did all the talking. On the other hand, Mel wasn't the sort of person you argued with . . . . what's that saying? Between a rock and a hard place or something!

It so happened that I had, a year or so before I met Mel, toyed with the idea of asking about being straightened up. I mentioned it to someone, I can't remember who, but whoever it was instantly, without pause, regaled me with tales of all of the . . . 'plegias I would get if I went ahead with this foolish notion, so I was discouraged. I weighed the life I had with AS progressing, against the risks of surgery, on balance I took the view that AS would be the lesser of the two evils.

I did nothing.

How though to respond to Mel, each week,

"Alan, we have it to do. Have you seen the doctor? What's he said? What did you say? Tell him he's an idiot" . . . . always a twinkle in her eye.

Often we sat and drank coffee in the break, she would tell me tales of what it is like to deliver a baby, what were her thoughts about being gay and thereby unlikely to have children and so it went, and, so did I, to my doctor. TM we will call him.

Dry mouthed, I sat in his room.

"Hi Alan. What can I do for you?"

"I want surgery on my spine, to straighten me up . . . . please."

"You are too old."

"Well I still want it."

"I am not sure if it can actually be done."

"Well will you find out?"

"Alan, this kind of surgery is very stressful, you are 42 and this is big stuff."

"Nevertheless, I would be grateful of you could find out for me."

Throughout this exchange, I had a vision of Mel in my mind, sat at coffee demanding to know the latest developments.

"Yes I will, I will refer you to the rheumatologist at the Queen's." (Queen's Medical Centre) and he did.

TM is a real person and my GP. He is, and has always been, a terrific doctor, supportive, willing and helpful. To his detriment though, it must be said that,

1. He hates Accordions and,
2. He sings in a Barber Shop Quartet!

The medical council though, still feel he is fit to practice . . . I owe him an enormous amount. Thank you so much Trevor.

Mel was thrilled to hear the tale and then immediately began to sit with someone else for coffee. Not as an affront to me but it was with a rather stunning looking other nurse, I think Mel quite liked her!

I was summoned to 'Harlow Wood' the spinal unit was based there, as I began this journey. It was switched to the Queen's fairly soon after. At this first visit, the stage was set for the coming metamorphosis.

John Webb the surgeon met me. He stood at the side of me.

"Stand up as straight as you can." he said.

"I am doing," I said.

His hand then pressed against my knees, the knees went back, the legs now straighter than for years, the shoulders neck and head tumbling forward and downward . . . .

"That's your real shape."

I was horrified.

"Imagine that you are at the side of a busy road and want to cross, keep your legs straight and look across this imaginary road."

Of course, I had no hope of looking across the road, imaginary or otherwise. I had a sudden and desperate cognisance of the real me, the grim enlightenment made more depressing by the knowledge that, as if this wasn't bad enough, it could and would get much worse.

J W then looked at me, straight in the face; my legs were bent again and head a little higher.

"What do YOU want ME to do?"

"I want you to straighten me up."

He made me tell him exactly what I wanted.

"Ok then, we will."

Wow . . . . was this really happening . . .

His two assistant doctors had been messing with me and drawing things on my back and, more importantly, on the life-size x-rays that had been taken that morning.

"What are you doing?" An icy tone.

"Well, we are trying to work out the angles."

"Well they are wrong. This is a spine you are dealing with, get the angles right."

It was a little embarrassing but I knew then that I was in very safe hands.

I was thrilled, elated. I knew that TM had come through for me, as he always does, and that they were going to do it. It is still impossible to describe the happiness I felt that day; I knew even then, that I had made a choice that would change my life forever.

I saw Mel the following Wednesday. She was back to taking coffee with me. I guessed that her overtures elsewhere were perhaps in the wrong key! I told her every detail.

She touched my elbow, smiled, "Super." she said, "Let me know everything as it happens."

Mel died suddenly, she was barely 50. Struck down from nowhere, sat at home after work and died. Mel never saw the results of my surgery, of which she was the instigator, the guide and the support.

Rest in Peace Mel x

I can't quite remember the name of that Finnish Javelin thrower. I recall that he was a huge man. He could hit a barn door at 9 miles. Little did I know that he worked part time on the spinal unit in Nottingham.

−Ten−

BACKING MY JUDGEMENT

I was summoned to the QMC a month later with instructions to take my lungs with me and at least one ear. Breathing was the thing and they were going to test it, but why, would one need an ear . . . .

Arriving in the lung functions department, I was introduced to a diminutive doctor, a specialist in lungs, I guessed. She was very pretty and petite. She was certainly working in the right department, for she took my breath away.

"Now Mr. Greaves," very formal and stiff,

"what we want to do is to hook you up to this machine, put this 12 inch diameter drainpipe inside your mouth, then we want you to ride a bicycle, fill in a form and pedal like there is no tomorrow!"

"The pipe will record your breathing rates when they change as you are pedalling."

I said nothing. Well it would have been difficult!! It was similar to a visit to the dentist, the kind of dentist who likes to insert 2 hands, a mirror, a cordless drill and a water suction pump into your mouth, some try to get their head in there as well, and then calmly say, "Hi Mr. Greaves, how are you today?"

Do they really expect an answer?

So there I am, practicing for the Tour de France, blowing hard into a small sewage pipe, when the large Finn sneaks up and sticks a javelin sized needle into my lobe. Now I knew why they wanted an ear. I looked at the doc imploringly trying with my eyes to say,

"Am I supposed to keep on pedalling or can I punch this geezer?"

In the meantime, blood was running freely from my ear, where a kind and fastidious nurse was making her best efforts to catch it in a bottle. The medical profession do seem to always have one at a disadvantage!!

Ear lobes bleed profusely, they are apparently the best place from which to take blood for the blood there is rich in oxygen. The purpose of all this was to see whether my system, (pulmonary, I think), could cope with the pressures that the impending surgery would place upon me. Like all spondylitics with a fused rib cage, breathing is easily compromised, 12 hours worth of anaesthesia to come would make those pressures severe.

Jan Zilezny, or something like that, yes, he was the Javelin man.

A week later I was told that lung functions were good and was given the ok to proceed to the next stage. I couldn't pass go, I certainly couldn't collect £200 yet, but the medical obstacles, that may impact on the agreement in principle to proceed with the surgery, were reduced by one.

I was counselled at length by the spinal team. Paralysis, loss of sexual ability, what not to do after the surgery, were some of the matters discussed as my possible future was laid out before me, and so it went.

My home telephone rang,

"Hi Alan, Jenny Sycamore here, don't get your hopes up, I'm not booking you in yet."

To explain, Jenny was the spinal ward manager, a tough cookie, but we got on ok.

"Alan"

"Yes Sister Sycamore."

"Alan I am just looking at your records, I see you are a smoker."

Bugger, I thought, this is going to stop everything.

"Oh well Sister, the lung function tests were ok."

"Oh it is alright Alan. I just wanted to say that you won't be smoking on or near my ward, will you Alan?"

Well what can one say when given a choice between not smoking, definitely not smoking, or absolutely not smoking at all?

"No Sister, no, well I have tried acupun . . . ."

The phone clicked and she was gone. The message, indelibly clear.

On the Monday following, I was in my workshop/office at the hotel with MA who was one of the hotel painters. I was taking a cigarette from my packet, MA was as well, our 8 o clock dizzy making drag long overdue,

"I'm fed up with smoking Mark."

"Me too Al."

"I'm giving up when I have finished this packet."

"Me too Al."

"Well I have said it often enough and I reckon I can do it this time."

"Me too Al."

"Right when I have finished this packet that's it, no more."

"Me too Al."

"Right, as of now I am a non-smoker."

"Me too Al."

Mark is a man of few words.

I had 3 in the packet, he had 17. It was by chance a busy day, so I got a cigarette in the lunch break and mid afternoon, this left one. I smoked it in the car on the way home, halfway through it I recalled my silly morning claim not to smoke again. I never have. Mark still does!

I was invited to Mark's wedding some years later, I said to him that I hoped all would go well for the future . . .

"Me too Al."

I was next summoned for the big tests, the ones to map brainwaves, the critical neurological stuff, to see if AS had damaged me so much that my responses to signals from the brain were impaired. The prospect of this troubled me, I wasn't on the operating table yet, would I get there?

A multi coloured plastic wig, a garden hosepipe and a lack of laxative would decide . . . .

A comedian was on stage at the gig, "I came here to do an impression of an idiot!" he said, "But you have beaten me to it! I told my son I would buy him a cowboy outfit for Christmas, so I bought him the Royal Hotel . . . ."

—Eleven—

BACK ON THE DOLE

In the meantime there was a bubbling sensation, growing, worrying, not in my body but at work. I worked for Queens Moat Houses, a large hotel chain mainly in England but with hotels in Europe too. Excellent hotels, ours in particular was spectacularly well run and making pots of money. The newspapers, when it broke, ran the headline:

"Second largest ever British business loss"

"2.8 billion in debt at Queens Moat Houses.

I was summoned again to the hospital shortly after this. Whilst there my head was wired with more than 50 cables, sandpaper used on the scalp to ensure secure glued fixings of each cable to my brainy nut. Wristlets were fixed together with straps around the ankles. Electrodes then at neck, shoulder, elbow, thigh and knee.

Laying on a bed, my makeshift wig stretching out above me (taking me well over 6 feet 5 for the first time in years), I was wheeled toward a computer where the fifty other ends of the cables were slowly, painstakingly connected to the input part of the machine. I wasn't worried, computers had taken men to the moon, not that I wanted this particular trip to end there!

All was set. On the bed, wires everywhere then one by one, charges were sent to each of the ankle and wristlets. It felt really odd. I found myself involuntarily giving the thumbs up sign with both hands, at the same time, simultaneously and together.!! There was nothing I could do to stop it.

I did think that restaurants might utilise this technology. "Did you enjoy your meal sir?" A waiters furtive grope and a surreptitious poke beneath the desk, then an unwilling thumb or two pop up, affirming that the meal was super dupe, whether in fact it was or not.

I digress, whilst all this was going on, a brainwave was visible on the monitor. This was kept and stored. Times were measured in terms of delay, from brain instruction to move thumb, to thumb actually moving. Later this information would become the most critical tool, other than the hammer and chisel used in the surgery.

Queens Moat board of directors were all removed bar one. A new team to head up the stricken group was selected by government officials and placed in charge. BA, the only former director remaining was awarded the unenviable task of sacking many hotel General Managers. Cruelly, whence he had completed this grim deed, he too was removed. A dirty trick.

We were untouched. Michael was the big boss and my friend, a man moving at a very different social level to me, a tough guy who seemed to like me. We always got on well and became good friends. (There is much to tell of Michael and the cruelty of fate, I have an empty space in my heart, but that is likely yet another tale for another day.) Michael explained at a meeting that he had had enough and would be moving on, he felt that others of us would be at risk too. He managed to secure a good voluntary redundancy deal for me.

I left the hotel, New Years Day, 1994.

In the meantime Jenny Sycamore had been busy and had let me know that all tests were now done, counselling complete, and everything was going ahead. It was all still quite unbelievable to me. I was sure that I would soon get a letter telling me that it had all been a ghastly mistake.

Did I want to proceed, she asked? Of course I did. Odd for me to be so determined on a course but in this case, the moment J. K. W. said they would do it, I never waivered (well nearly never, there was that one moment!) from the pathway to surgery.

I said a sad goodbye to Michael and others at the Royal. I had enjoyed great times there, the job had put me well on to enjoying life without drink, put money in my pocket and stimulated my intellectual desires. I had loved the Royal, so left with a heavy heart, but knew that when Michael left the following month, that it would never be the same again.

I used the redundancy money to build a small workshop at the side of my house. I had a plan.

Jenny rang me in March, the date had been set . . . . May 14th . . . .

How odd is the formulation, the timing of life's chapters, a happy time at the Royal ending, a huge door opening toward something that may be wonderful or terrible . . . . I had a cup of tea . . . . the hosepipe next.

Part 3

The telling time, the time of my life, the right time, just in time!

–Twelve–

I arrived at the hospital on Tuesday morning, not a long drive, just 2 miles from home, on the same road in fact. I was looking for Ward D8 west block. The Queen's Medical Centre is large, very large, a hideously designed building externally, but ok inside. I had concerns that it would take me forever to find where I needed to be. I was a little uptight, I had not been an in-patient for some years and never at the Queen's. Thus I was uncertain as to how it would go. I found the main reception desk.

"Excuse me could you direct me to ward D8 West block please, is it far?"

"Get in the lift there, go up 2 floors, go in the door facing the lift and you are there."

Wow, and it was. This had all been so easy, a good omen I thought.

"Hello my name is Alan Greaves, I am booked in for surgery."

"You're early." She shot at me, an accusation almost.

"Ahh well you see the traff . . . ." I stumbled.

Then she smiled, "No its ok, your bed is ready, you are in Blue Six."

My anxieties had caused me to misinterpret her manner.

"I'll fetch Sister Sycamore."

As she spoke, I saw the formidable personage of Jenny Sycamore bustling around the corner just ahead of me, moving swiftly in my direction. The staff in that instant, to a man and a woman, became very busy!

"Hi Alan, lovely to see you, have you booked in?"

"Was just doing so."

"Ok, I'll make you a cuppa."

Wow she was lovely and whilst she was clearly the boss, she had a gentle nature.

"Oh Jenny," I chanced my arm with her Christian name, "Jenny, I stopped smoking."

I smugly awaited the congratulations that were rightly my due. She looked at me and smiled.

"Oh I knew you would." she said, and headed to the tea room.

I sat with a nursing auxiliary on the bed at Blue Six, a small ward of six beds, two rows of three, facing each other. Mine was on the end nearest the corridor. How useful that would turn out to be!

I filled in all sorts of forms, signed all sorts of forms, filled in more forms, had a blood test, was weighed, urine sample given, temperature and all the usual stuff. It was a wonderfully relaxed routine. Surgery was definitely scheduled for next morning. All forms satisfactorily filled, I asked the auxiliary if I was now to get into bed. I sort of expected that I would need to be pyjama-clad and goody goody-ishly tucked up, ready for Matrons visit.

"Bugger off to the canteen."

"Oh," Somewhat taken aback.

"Straight down the corridor at the end."

So I did.

There, a pair of peculiar things happened. One, I remember, was walking along the corridor when a smartly dressed man walked towards me. He stared at me. For some reason I was walking full stoop, I had neglected to do the knees bend trick, I felt this man swivel and stare at me as we passed by each other. I felt sure that he stared at me all during my journey along the corridor.

In another room, a man was selling books, young good looking.

I had a sandwich, then went to the ward once more . . . .

"Ahhh where have you been?"

"Canteen as I was told."

"Well we have forms to fill in."

I assured them that I had done myriad forms but was told no, there were some more.

Time was moving into the afternoon by now so I sat and read a while.

My wife and young daughters visited early evening. I was visited too and at the same time by the anaesthetist.

"Can we see Dad tomorrow?" Asked Ruth.

"Oh errr . . . mmmmmm. well, err tell you what Ruth, perhaps it would be better if you leave it a few days because Dad might be quite tired!"

This was my first indication that this was not going to be entirely an easy ride. Rufus was upset. Esther, my youngest, ever the pragmatist, was helping herself to my lemonade and a chocolate biscuit. She has always had a capacity for identifying the more important matters.

My family left, wishing me luck and promising to be there, well, Ellen-my wife would be.

Alone now with the anaesthetist, a down to earth man, he asked if he could do an experiment during the surgery.

Normally, before these things, not to put too fine a point on it, one is drowned in laxative to empty the system. He didn't want to do this, he preferred to insert a tube through the nose into the gut and stop the gut working, then take noxious fluids away via the tube.

"It will be ok, we will insert it when you are under the anaesthetic."

This was slightly reassuring.

"Ok."

Later this would seem not to have been my best decision in life; to choose the tube again or being trapped under a hotel shutter, what a dilemma.

Chris Cain then came by.

"Alan you will feel some pain when you wake from the surgery, in the legs."

"Oh that's fine, I didn't expect it all to be easy, I will cope."

He gave me a knowing smile. He then drew out on an envelope precisely what he/they would be doing, and drills, hammers, chisels, screwdrivers, spoons and much other equipment would be used.

"See you in the morning then Alan."

A very nice man.

A hint of disquiet had come upon me, what with tubes, Dad being 'tired' to keep my girls away from possible distress, pains after the surgery, then a rethink over the months of tests and counselling. I think, be it at the eleventh hour, I was beginning to understand that when T M described this as 'Big Surgery' he meant 'BIG' surgery.

It finally dawned upon me that I was taking enormous risk and that my usually happy outlook, may be severely tested in the very near future.

Jenny appeared, she seemed almost to live there.

"You are first in Alan because you will be in all day, so up at 5 in the morning, shower, bathroom, then the technician will wire your head."

I was alone in bed now, thought to do a crossword but found that I couldn't concentrate. I slept not at all that night. I wondered. Who was the odd man who had stared at me in the corridor? Why couldn't Rufus see me the next day? Why was the theatre booked for the whole day? All in all, I was in a euphoric state not quite believing that this was all happening, but less cheery thoughts were beginning to form deeper in my mind, however, I shook myself, dispelling the small gloomy cloud that had descended upon me. Wouldn't it be marvellous; home in a few days, tall, lovely . . . . AS though, even when retreating from skilled surgeons would soon find ways of letting me know it was still there, live and kicking. Four a.m. arrived. I needed not to be awoken. I wandered to the bathroom and errrr . . . couldn't. A horrid thought hit me, what if I do on the operating table, god I hoped not. The Neurology technician arrived. There were only two articulated lorries full of cables, well there were so many it seemed that way. It took her two hours to wire me up, then a porter arrived. J. K. W. made an appearance, he grabbed my big toe.

"Morning Alan, ready?"

I was wheeled to the elevators, taken up I think, then wheeled what felt like miles to the theatre suite, the Anaesthetist awaited me; he held a large garden hosepipe in his hand.

"Is that it? It's a bit bigger than I expected."

"Don't worry you'll be asleep."

Chris Cain, dressed in theatre blues, protective spectacles, hat and everything, walked past me, touching my arm.

"You ready then Alan?"

"Yes."

I felt a ticking in my left arm; the anaesthetic was going in; a clock on the wall in front and above me said 6:57 a.m.

Fear, terrible fear gripped me.

"What am I doing here, God will I be ok?"

Then, I was back in bed, not that I knew where I was, who I was or what I was; I only knew that I was screaming.

I have no experience of drug taking for recreational purposes. My brother was a heroin addict, he died, too young. He was 56. I miss him.

—Thirteen—

IS MY BACK, BACK?

I was full of morphine (as such, much of what I write now is based upon all that I was told after the events). At my moment of waking I was incapable of thought. I had no awareness of who or where I was. A sense within me kept saying that something was wrong, desperately wrong. But what was wrong? I had no idea for I had no idea of what anything was.

A 4 inch by 4 inch square appeared before me, it had vertical stripes of various greens, I knew this square, well didn't know it, but deep within I knew that this square meant something to me. It disappeared. It came and went many times. It hovered around, butterfly like in its flickering movement. What was it?

My face hurt and had something sticky all over it. I was trying to push it off but each time I did so it was there on my face again. My right forefinger hurt and felt squashed. I was tied down and could touch the ropes that contained me. The square reappeared. It waivered in front of me and then was gone, what was this square, I should know this square! I yelled out and was engulfed in pain, pain far worse than that, that I have known all of my adult life. This pain wouldn't go away, I couldn't get into a position where I might relieve it a little. My finger felt funny, what was this sticky thing over my face. Then noises, then the square, then the pain then the noise then the square and the pain. It went on, day after day.

My mind reeled, I began to have thoughts, or what I believed might be thoughts, but they were jumbled, incomprehensible, but important to me to understand them. Will it be best to keep pyjamas on underneath my suit or best to keep suit under pyjamas, I couldn't decide which would be easier, if I keep my suit under my pyjamas, I can get to work easier, but then what about bedtime, no perhaps pyjamas over my suit will be easier so when I have finished work I can go back to hospital and get into bed!

I don't want a shave, I can shave myself. Green square, Hilary shouting, hold his head, scrape, scrape as the blade shuddered across my face. I don't want a shave, the green square, steady now in front of me, pain, screaming, tearful pain, pain, pain. Who was I, what was happening to me.

And so it went. Morphine is not fun, it plays with the mind, and yet without it what would that pain have been like? I had somehow worked out that 4 days had passed, I had realised who I was, where I was and even why I was there. I knew then that I was ok. I understood somehow that 4 days had passed and I was OK. The green square became a little bigger.

"Look at yourself, look at yourself."

It could talk.

"He's taken that clip off his finger again."

I heard it in the far distance. Someone squashed my finger.

"Will he leave that mask on."

"Alan, now leave the mask, it will help you breathe."

"I don't want it."

"Alan, hold this button, now if it hurts, just press the button. It will give you some morphine and stop the pain."

I pressed the button as if I was competing in the world button pressing championships, the pain continued, unabated.

This went on for hours. I wanted to be dead. I didn't want to be here and didn't want to be whoever I was.

I was in the HDU ward (High Dependency Unit)

I had been there only 2 hours, not 4 days.

"Look at yourself, look at yourself."

It was the next day. I had spent twenty-four agonising, sleepless hours in unstoppable agony. I begged for it to stop.

The green square appeared, it was attached to other green squares which formed a blouse that my wife was wearing. She had been there all the time.

"Look at yourself" she said.

"I don't want to effing look at myself, if I had known what it was going to be like, I would never have had it done, you just don't understand."

Yes I actually spoke those silly and selfish words. To this day I can hear myself saying them and looking at Ellen, crushed by my cruelty. I regretted it immediately, even through the morphine haze, the pain, that bloody mask stuck to my face, I knew I had been selfish and hurtful. Sadly, I wasn't able to formulate apologetic words for the mental capacity wasn't there; I think to this day that that comment sits between us.

Day two and I was alert now, and because I was alert realised just how much pain I was in. They were reducing the morphine, so my brains were slowly returning. Another shave from Hilary, a rather cool mannered humourless nurse, efficient though and capable.

Then, two physiotherapists were appointed to attend upon me and life got a whole lot worse. I think it was two mornings later, maybe it was three, my memory tricks me nowadays. A lovely young lady and her even younger male assistant, the physiotherapists, arrived at my bedside. They were both similarly attired in cheery smiles, enthusiastically demonstrating a 'here to help' attitude.

"Right Alan, can you stand up for us please."

I was horror-struck. "I can't even lie down for you." I croaked.

"All right then Alan, you stay there then, now let's just move these blankets over here."

She opened my pyjama jacket and spread it wide, exposing the white rather charmless opaque and fleshy chest beneath.

She placed both hands on top of my chest, palms down with fingers spread wide.

"Alan, now I want you to cough for me please, nice and hard, we need to clear this anaesthetic and get your lungs working."

Well I felt grim and I hurt like hell but thought, well, she only wants me to cough, so I did.

Now I really screamed. It is difficult to explain, unless you have been in a similar situation, what a simple cough can do. I made an attempt at a fairly vigorous expectoration, not fully appreciating the engineering involved. I breathed deeply, slowly, drawing as much air as possible into lungs which were and are captive beneath a ribcage which has entirely fused. These self same ribs, by chance, were attached to a fused spine, the very spine in fact which had so very recently been drilled, chopped, screwed, glued, opened and closed, broken and subject to goodness knows how much other random D.I.Y. The cough and the energy in it, rocketed down to the operation site. The pain was just, well, beyond all that I have already described in these pages. Short lived thankfully and I immediately realised that if I didn't cough (I learn quickly when pain is in the offing), I wouldn't have to bear that particularly exquisite agony again.

"Oh Alan that was really good," hands spread once more, "now can we (we??) do one more?"

No, no, not again, I cringed away from them as far as the mattress would allow, which was not far enough.

"Now Alan you really must, just to make sure your lungs are clear."

I thought to humour her and attempted a throat clearing noise which I tried to dress up as a cough.

"Ok Alan yes, we will do some more tomorrow."

"You won't," I thought, but was relieved that they had done . . . hadn't they?

"Right Alan. Right, let's see if we can stand you up and take a few steps."

I didn't know what to do.

Next thing I was log rolled slowly and carefully, sideways across the bed so that my feet were on the floor and the top corner of the side of the bed behind my knees.

So far so good. The young fellow took one of my arms, the girl the other, a brief scream, an agonising but mercifully short pain at the operation site and I was on my feet. I felt that a round of applause might be appropriate but was denied such plaudits. Next they let go of me, mistake, a terrifying mistake, I knew at that moment that I was not going to survive. I was toppling backwards, in the manner of a recently felled tree; a slow, inexorable, languorous backwards fall, tall, rigid, unable to help my self. They managed to grab my arms, to my amazement and relief, I landed almost where I had started, flat and across the bed, and they managed to make it a soft landing. The only pain was that of fear, had I broken my spine? Had the wound been opened? Had the rods come adrift? What if a rogue screw was now positioned beneath my heart just waiting to pierce me for good and all. But, I was ok.

Thankfully they fairly quickly 'log rolled' me back into bed where I was left alone for a while.

I didn't realize it but I was covered in tubes, the aforementioned garden hose was still inserted, there were drains in the wound, with other odd things in my mouth and ears, a line through the neck directly into the heart, a catheter, lines into both hands; this was the cause of the tied down vision I had had on the first day. A pulse taking clip was on my finger and I still had to wear an oxygen mask.

The weather was very hot. This was unfortunate and did add somewhat to the general feeling of discomfort.

By now I was seeing visitors, (not my children), even Ellen didn't want them to see me yet. I must have looked a fearful sight. I was beginning to really unscramble the morphine mix in my brain. Sufficient to say that, as ever, the pain was severe, ever present.

'Log rolling' was essential, if it were mistimed even ever so slightly, rarely for they were a superb team, it was agonising. I wasn't managing to eat, even my beloved tea was impossible to get down.

The staff nurse, a chap called Jim, was concerned about the warmth. He positioned a floor standing fan at the foot of my bed. It was lovely. I basked in the cool flowing air, smug about mine being the only one provided.

I had not been to the bathroom yet. You will recall that I had a few days before, on the morning of the surgery, been unable. My gut wasn't working, it hadn't switched on yet.

The following morning I felt as dreadful as I ever have in all of my life. I had a severe chill, no gut, in pain, no nourishment. So, so poorly did I feel that they rang Ellen and asked her to come to see me earlier than was usual.

'F and M', my own music teachers and long standing family friends, came to visit. I lay there unable to communicate. I was ashamed and felt that I had been unacceptably rude to them.

I was unable to sleep, pain, pain, pain, and really thought what a complete and vain idiot I had been to do this. I was going to pay a real price for it and I didn't care, I just wanted someone to flick a switch and turn me off. Oh to be free of this mess.

Ellen was in distress, I could see it, even through my self pity.

I slept all night.

I awoke at 6 a.m. log rolled myself onto the edge of the bed, stood and walked to the bathroom. How I did it I don't know, only that I did. Without dwelling too much on unnecessary, less pleasant matters, I was in there for nearly an hour because it was shall we say, challenging! The nature of this activity places pressure on the spine, and so was very painful. A nurse came in, in the end and helped me back to bed.

I felt so dammed good.

Ellen rang the ward sister, sobbing, convinced that she would be told the worst. The sister brought the phone to me, we chatted, Ellen was disbelieving,

"I thought you were going to die."

"So did I, I think it was the loo that did it! Will you bring me some lemonade and a crossword book please?"

One corner had been turned. There was worse to come, the leg pains referred to on the eve of the surgery decided to come a calling, 'leg pains' was then and remains a wholly inadequate description. The turtle impression was yet to happen and Ellen walked me up the ward where she knew there was a full length mirror.

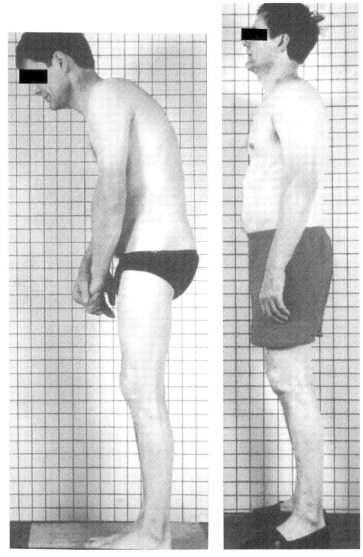

A dramatic view of before and after. Remember that the before picture is 2 years prior to surgery, I was bent even further forward at the time of the surgery.

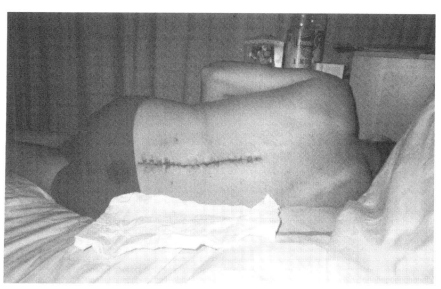

Mirror, mirror on the wall, who is the straightest and so tall?
Lemonade ever present!

—Fourteen—

Back To Normality, Nearly

The man from the corridor appeared at my bedside. He grinned rather inanely at me.

"I saw you the other day, in the corridor."

"Yes, yes I remember."

"I can't believe this. I have never ever seen this."

I looked at him, enquiringly.

"This surgery, I remember you from the corridor, how bent over you were, now you are straight, this is amazing, I have never seen this before."

He must have realised my confusion, for his face lit up, he grinned and told me who he was and why he was at my bedside.

"Oh Alan, yes, to explain. I am C W, I am an orthopaedic surgeon from California. I am doing a fellowship with Mr. W., I was in theatre during your surgery."

I now understood. He explained how he had noticed me on the corridor and seen that I was spondylitic. He was excited because he realised that I was the one to undergo the procedure that he had come to learn about; it was also the biggest surgery he had ever been involved in. He was quite overcome by it all, thrilled at the 'before and after'.

We chatted a good while, he told me a remarkable story.

"I work in a partnership of three orthopaedic surgeons in California.

One of my partners has AS, he looks as you looked a few days ago. We have never seen this procedure."

He was clearly, obviously stunned at the procedure and its results.

"I am going to bring my partner to England to undergo this procedure."

A compliment indeed. Whether he brought his partner over to England or not, I don't know. He took away two pre-op pictures that I gave to him.

J. W. and Chris Cain arrived early one morning. J. W. explained that the spondylitic actions which had caused me to need surgery, would immediately start the bending process again. Surgery was wonderful but of course the AS was still present and continuing on with its dirty deeds. I had to remain as upright as possible, particularly, if you will forgive the pun, straight after surgery.

He/they proposed to put me into a plaster jacket that day. The Orthotist arrived in the afternoon. I was taken by wheelchair into his room. I then had to stand and he began the process of sealing me up. Here I encountered my first problem. I hadn't stood unsupported for more than a few moments at a time. I could walk a little but standing still, with arms akimbo, so that he could get the bandages beneath them, was impossible; my legs shook with pain and exhaustion. The Orthotist allowed me to take breaks and sit whilst he measured and cut and trimmed. The other, and later, more serious problem, was that sitting was the most painful of all postures. The plastering process was tiring, agonizing, long winded and particularly uncomfortable.

Eventually, I was done. I now had a carapace, an external skeleton, it was awful, I hated it instantly. My already limited comfort was now impinged upon beyond any hope of relief.

I was assisted into bed, I still needed to be log rolled, suddenly this simple activity, performed by a minimum of two nurses took on a scary new dimension. With one nurse at legs, the other at shoulders, the idea was to roll me over in absolute unison; if legs were behind shoulders and vice versa, the result was a twist in the lumbar spine, in other words, agony.

The plaster jacket made it an impossible job for the nurse at the shoulders, she was unable to judge precisely whether I was moving inside the jacket at the right pace. I was severely twisted at the operation site twice that evening.

My family arrived, my girls too, it was so fabulous to see them.

"Dad, have you any biscuits left?"

"Dad can I have some lemonade please?"

It was marvellous to see and hear them. It was wonderful to see that their lives had their own special important bits, lemonade and biscuits, what an excellent prescription for a pair of lovely girls. They all laughed at me propped by now in the large chair at the side of the bed.

"Dad you look like a tortoise."

"Dad, can I write on the plaster please?"

It was a lovely evening. It passed by far too quickly. I was fairly soon helped into bed by Ellen and the nurses since the chair was not at all comfortable.

Lying down on your back in a shell-like plaster is weird and a touch scary. I was unable to move, I felt utterly trapped. I hated this thing, it had been on for a mere few hours, I had to wear it for 6 months. I was really concerned that I would not be able to get through it.

I was assisted out of bed and went to the toilet, another novel experience!

Some weeks later my wife explained to me, a small incident that occurred on the way home from that visit. She had already explained to the girls about the tubes and that Dad looked a bit of a mess. When they arrived, the only tube remaining was the catheter. A catheter is tiny in diameter at the insertion end but the tube then, in an increasing taper, becomes around an inch in diameter. Ruth was fascinated by this; the only visible part of course was the one inch section. On the bus home she asked Mum to confirm that this particular tube was in Dad's 'willy'! Oh yes, said Mum.

"Wow, Mum, Dad must have a giant 'willy'."

Modesty obliges me to refrain from comment.

—Fifteen—

FROM BACK TO WORSE

Walking back to the bed, Chris Cain's 'leg pains' hit me. A sudden spasm in the back of the hip, so excruciating that I (yes again) screamed but in terror realised that I was face down on the floor and bellowing like a baby. The nursing cavalry arrived poste haste. Jenny Sycamore, reassuring as ever, directed operations and I was raised from the floor and carried to bed. Once flat on the bed and all were breathing a little easier, spasm 2 hit me and this was twice as bad as the first. Stan in Blue Three woke up and yelled at me to shut up. I was very rude to him, which I must say is entirely unlike me. Then spasm number 3. By spasm number 4, I was peculiarly positioned with my left foot on the floor, my right leg on the bed and the rest of me somewhere between, held precariously in place by 2 nurses. There were 23 spasms that night. Without question it was the most agonising night of my life, then and now. As I sit and type this, I remember every spasm, every word from every nurse. I use the word 'Grim' too much but this night was truly as grim as could be.

Morphine by the gallon was administered. Eventually I collapsed into fitful and grateful sleep. Next morning CC was there first thing.

"Alan it's coming off today, do you need anything?"

A smiling thank you and a huge sigh of relief flooded over through and within me.

"No, not at the moment thanks."

The Orthotist arrived, he removed the tortoiseshell. It had been in place for less than 24 hours . . . . thank God.

The battle wasn't over yet, the spasms hadn't disappeared, but I did get a nice new jacket out of the deal.

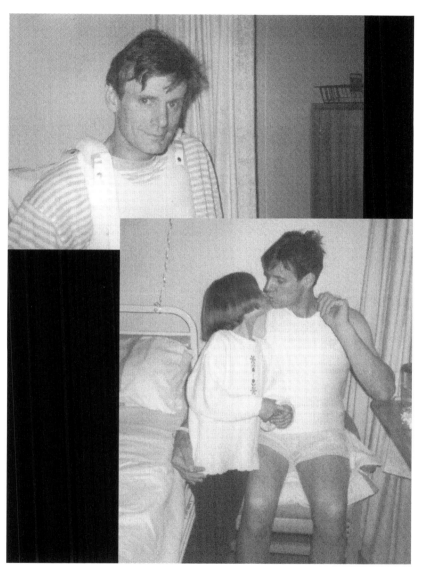

Night, night Esther!

I wish that I could see my back
To look it up and down
I wish I didn't have a back
That makes me look a clown

I wish I had, a spine that was
Bendy soft yet strong
That needs no rods no screws inside
To stop it going wrong.

-Sixteen-

BACK INSIDE THE LOOKING GLASS

"Look at yourself, look."

I stood in front of a full length mirror, side on with head turned to my right. There was a straight tall man looking back at me. Was it me? Goodness, it can't be, but it was. The stress of the surgery melted away. I stood humbled, looking at the evidence of the disappearance of years and years of staring at the floor. It quite took my breath away.

"Look, see, I told you. Look."

I just stood and looked, I couldn't talk, couldn't respond to Ellen.

It had worked. I wasn't paralysed, it had worked. The joy in me was restrained, held back, never one really for a dramatic public showing of honest, 'how I felt' drama. The joy in me was palpable, it was quietly overwhelming. I was overwhelmingly quiet. I stood and stared at the new me.

I loved the new me.

As we walked away, I couldn't help but feel that I was falling over; backwards. So many years hunched over and suddenly I felt that I was leaning backwards.

Muscles that had been constrained, limited for years were now free to flex and move. I could get rid of indigestion so easily! My legs could walk and stand straight and I could see across the road. This was not an instant happiness, more of a growing, glowing one that became ever headier as I discovered one by one, all of the new things, the ordinary things that I could do.

I was wearing my new Velcro fastening plastic jacket. This was a compromise, it acted as the plaster would have done, but I could adjust this one and more to the point, I could remove it. If I was going to walk, I put it on and tightened it pretty well as tight as it could be. Sitting and I could wear it slightly looser. For sleeping, then it stood on the floor at the side of my bed, a disembodied torso shining white in the night.

Spasms were almost a regular part of getting out of and into bed. The positioning of every part of me had to be precise and the timing too. Sometimes I could rise from the bed quite easily. Getting back in was many times more difficult and it was usually then that I endured the really strong spasms. By now I had been in the hospital for two weeks. I wanted to be away home.

"Will I be discharged this week Jenny?"

"If I discharged you, could you manage at home Alan?"

"Errr, well . . . ."

"Err nothing, you know you couldn't, go and have a cuppa."

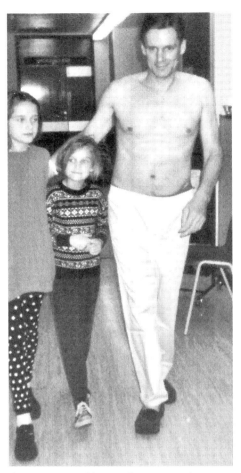

See the operating table anywhere? Hi Rufus x, Hi Es x!

I was receiving anti-rejection injections daily. Apparently some peoples bodies reject the titanium instrumentation, the skin goes black and rots, this was a worry because the only way to deal with rejection is to open up the operation site and remove the rods and screws. No, I couldn't face that, thus, I was grateful that I again was lucky and showed no signs of rejection.

The day that I had asked to be discharged, in the afternoon, Jenny came to me and asked if I would mind if a man came to see me the next day. He too had AS and was contemplating similar surgery. Would I chat with him about the whole experience?

The man arrived the next day. He was older than me and also had Parkinson's Disease. He was quite stooped. His wife was with him. Jenny brought them to me and then left us to it.

I talked and answered questions, much along the lines of these foregoing rather random chapters. The man's wife said, "No, No you aren't having it." The man seemed to nod assent. When I saw Jenny some time after, she told me that the man had decided against surgery, it was too much to go through.

Perhaps it was.

There were many more worrying moments, more wonderful care, a staff of doctors and nurses who were second to none. I won't go into every detail here, sufficient to say I was on the mend.

I went home after 3 and a half weeks in hospital, I still couldn't sit or lay down alone but I more or less insisted that I go. Jenny was still not thrilled with the idea. As soon as I was home I was in big trouble, night times a living hell, my family wonderful.

Ellen was popping next door and left Esther babysitting me!

"Mum, what shall I do if Dad screams?"

"Just ignore him."

Ellen was gone for nearly 5 minutes so Esther was spared such decision making.

Five weeks later I went for a walk to watch Rufus in her school sports day. I was very tired and in pain when I got there. Neither were there chairs so I stood. Walking back home was agonising, though somewhat defraying the misery was Ruth's proud smirk and purple 'pinned on ribbon' for second place in the egg and spoon race.

From that day, the spasms and the night pain stopped. The very worst was over. It was one year later however, before I could contemplate the thought of a return to work. AS seemed to take pity on me during that year and was relatively un-troublesome.

When I went back to work I soon realised that I had made a mistake. I battled on for 12 months as a construction site joiner, then a maintenance joiner but knew that my time 'On the tools' was over, I couldn't do it anymore. I felt that each moment of the day would bring a wrong move that would undo all the good that had been done in my name.

I eventually took a job in an office where I have become overweight and again wracked with the pains of AS; I have in the last 2 years bent forward over the top of my rods by nearly 12 inches. AS back in full swing.

I am now under the care of a super Rheumatologist Dr Ira Pande. She has given me the opportunity to try out a biological drug (Enbrel-Etanercept). It works, it reduces the pain very well. Unfortunately I have so much mechanical damage throughout my skeletal structure that it works only on new inflammation. I can only wonder what my life would have been like had these drugs been available many years ago, however, it doesn't matter. Dr IP looks after me so very well and has given me real improvement and optimism. She, like all the other teams that have looked after me, are the heroes of this tale.

In the Police Force 40 years ago I have written that I was in terrible pain, today the pain is the same. AS is a cruel master, it has bent me to its will, I am what I am because of it, but odd to say, I would not have missed the experiences it has brought to me, not for the world.

I am one of the lucky ones, blessed to live in a town where spinal care is supreme. Blessed by the many Doctors who have given of themselves for me, and continue to do so. Blessed because through them, all of them, my life continues to be worthwhile and exciting and purposeful.

Fifteen years later, I am tall and strong, life is new and wonderful.

I am one of life's rare and privileged people.

Years of Ankylosing Spondylitis and then the surgery has taken my life to unexpected places. All of those experiences make me what I am, I am happy to be me.

-Seventeen-

MY BACK IN THEATRE

So what is the fuss about, why was this difficult surgery, what did they actually do?

Essentially, the human spine is a spring, a spring, which is long and shaped like a letter 'S'.

Ankylosing Spondylitis destroys the joints which make the spine springy and bendy. In my case the spine had/has no joints or disc pads. It does not twist, bend or lean. It is affected from hips to skull. In brief, AS had turned my spine into a large single slab of bone, twice its normal diameter with no spinal functionality at all. The Lumbar section, 'the small of the back' which would normally house the lower part of the 'S' shape had become straight and it was this that forced the top half of the spine to bend forward so dramatically.

The surgeon's objective was to re-form a curve into the lumbar spine. If successful, this would reverse some of the bending affect at the top of the spine.

Two wedges were chiselled out of lumbar vertebrae 2 and 4. (See illustration below). The remainder of the chiselled joints were then snapped. The spinal cord was exposed by the removal of processes and pedicles—snapped off with pliers. Bone was harvested from the left hip. All of the removed bony material was stored.

The spine was then manipulated into its new shape. When surgeons were happy with the shape, they formed 2 rods of Titanium into the same contour. These were then screwed to the spine on either side to hold the spine in its new shape. During this part of the procedure the spinal cord, which for years had been distorted to the shape of the diseased spine, was put carefully into its new shape. The bruising caused by touching the spinal cord during this procedure was the cause of the previously described agonising spasms.

Harvested and stored bone matter was then glued back in to the spine. This would protect the cord and grow into the spine to lock it in its new shape.

How?

Holes were drilled either side of each vertebra that was to be broken. The spinal vertebral body has a hard outer shell but the material inside is softer honeycomb type material. Special spoons were inserted through the drilled holes and the vertebra hollowed out. A chisel was then carefully placed at the required angle and the outer shell chopped away.

All very simple then!!!

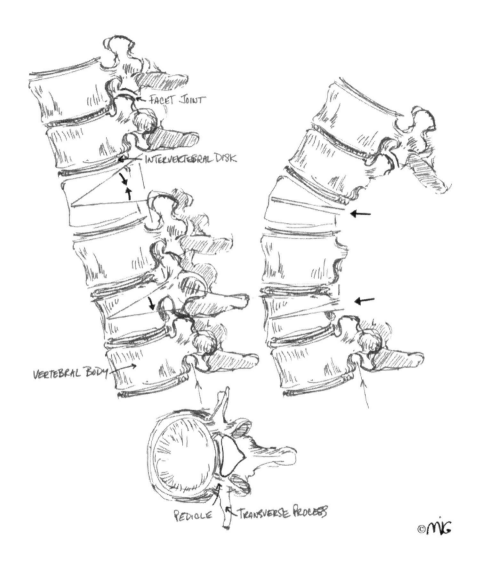

FACET JOINT

INTERVERTEBRAL DISK

VERTEBRAL BODY

PEDICLE

TRANSVERSE PROCESS

©MG

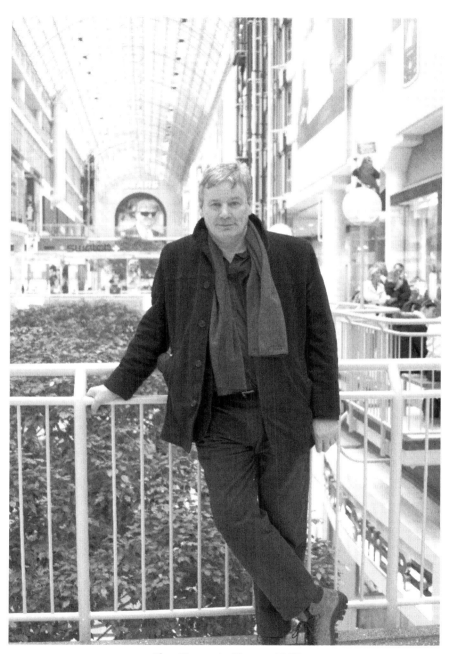

Alan Greaves in Toronto 2007

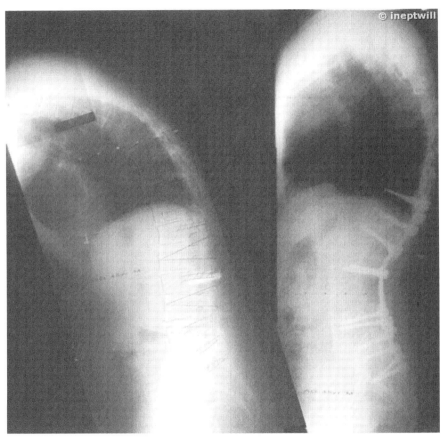

A dramatic before and after x-ray. Note the thickness of the spine and the lack of joints. An ironmonger's delight!

So many grateful thanks:

To my friends Colin and Mig who encouraged me to write.

To the Queens Medical Centre team.

In gratitude for a debt that I can never repay

To

Trevor Mills—John Webb—Chris Cain—Jenny Sycamore

For Mel and

In remembrance of my friend

Michael Slagle

In grateful thanks for the ongoing care and skills of

Dr Ira Pande

To

My wife, my children, my parents, my sister and brothers.

Thank you all, for doing so very much for me.

AG—2009.

Epilogue-

I have said that 2 things happened during my first walk to the hospital canteen. One was CW the surgeon staring at me, the other, a man selling books.

As a present to me for undergoing this surgery, because books are precious, my wife purchased a book from this man, 'Hutchinson's Encyclopaedia'.

Some time after my surgery I met my son whom I had not seen for 20 years.

He sells books for a living, he visits church halls and hospitals and the like. He has sold a lot of Hutchinson's. He sold one to a woman at the Queens Medical Centre in May 1994

He remembered that it was a gift for her husband, who had undergone some surgery . . . !

Gone straight at last!